Digestive Range: "Navigating the Digestive System for Optimal Health"

Dolores E. Flint

Digestive Range: "Navigating the Digestive System for Optimal Health"

Disclaimer:

Table of Contents

Chapter 8: Dietary and Lifestyle Guidelines to Support Digestive Health

Conclusion

INTRODUCTION

The human digestive system is a marvel of complexity, coordinating the digestion, absorption, and utilization of nutrients required for survival. From the moment food enters the mouth until the waste is evacuated, this complicated system goes through a series of highly tuned processes that are critical to our life and well-being. However, despite its critical role, gut health is frequently disregarded until symptoms emerge. In this complete guide to digestive health, we will take a tour through the gastrointestinal tract's structure, functions, and the many elements that influence its overall health. We look at how gut health affects not just physical energy but also mental and emotional equilibrium. Throughout this book, we will look at the mechanics behind common digestive illnesses such as irritable bowel syndrome (IBS), acid reflux, inflammatory bowel disease (IBD), and more. Understanding the underlying causes and triggers of these disorders allows us to make more informed health decisions and seek suitable treatment and management options. Furthermore, we will investigate the symbiotic relationship between nutrition and digestive health, determining how our food choices influence the operation of our gastrointestinal tract. From the function of fiber in encouraging regularity to the impact of probiotics on gut flora, we'll look at the dietary concepts that promote healthy digestion and general health. Beyond nutrition, we will look at the impact of lifestyle factors like stress, exercise, and sleep on gut health. Recognizing the interdependence of mind and body allows us to employ holistic ways that promote digestive health and improve our quality of life. Throughout this book, we hope to give you practical information and concrete solutions for improving your digestive health. Whether you want to relieve digestive discomfort, prevent future problems, or simply improve your general well-being, this guide will be a great help on your journey to digestive wellness.

Join us on a journey through the digestive tract, understanding the secrets of the stomach and enabling ourselves to nourish, care, and cherish our bodies' inner landscape.

Chapter 1: Anatomy of the Digestive System

The digestive system is a complex network of organs and tissues that combine to digest food, absorb nutrients, and eliminate waste. From the moment food enters the mouth until it is expelled as waste, this complicated system goes through a series of synchronized actions to extract vital nutrients and energy for the body's survival.

• **Mouth:** The digestive process begins in the mouth, where food is swallowed and chewed, resulting in smaller particles. Saliva, generated by salivary glands, includes enzymes that start the breakdown of carbohydrates.

• **Esophagus:** After chewing and mixing with saliva, food goes down the esophagus, which is a muscular tube that connects the throat to the stomach. Peristaltic waves help force food downward, a process known as swallowing.

• **Stomach:** In the stomach, food is further broken down by stomach acid and enzymes, resulting in a semi-liquid material known as chyme. The stomach lining secretes gastric fluids, such as hydrochloric acid and pepsin, to aid in protein digestion.

• **Small Intestine:** The small intestine absorbs the vast majority of nutrients. It is separated into three parts: the duodenum, jejunum, and ileum. The pancreas' enzymes and the liver's bile help break down carbs, proteins, and lipids into their component components for absorption into the bloodstream.

The large intestine (colon) absorbs water and electrolytes, resulting in excrement. The colon also contains a large colony of helpful bacteria known as the gut microbiota, which aids digestion, nutrition absorption, and immunological function.

• **Rectum and Anus:** Feces are kept in the rectum and released from the body via the anus during defecation.

Peristalsis, or smooth muscular contractions, drives food and waste products along the digestive tract. Digestion is closely regulated by a complex combination of hormones, neurons, and feedback mechanisms that maintain adequate nutrition absorption and waste disposal.

Understanding the anatomy of the digestive system reveals how the body properly processes food and maintains life. By nurturing and supporting this complex system through appropriate dietary and lifestyle choices, we can improve gut health and overall well-being.

Chapter 2: Understanding Digestive Disorders

Understand Digestive Disorders

Digestive disorders are a broad category of illnesses that affect the gastrointestinal tract, affecting normal function and causing discomfort, pain, and other symptoms. Understanding these illnesses is critical for efficient management and therapy, whether they are minor symptoms like indigestion or chronic conditions like inflammatory bowel disease (IBD). Here's a summary of several major digestive disorders:

• **Gastroesophageal Reflux Disease (GERD):** GERD is caused by stomach acid flowing back into the esophagus, resulting in irritation and inflammation. Heartburn, regurgitation, chest pain, and difficulty swallowing are among the possible symptoms.

• **Peptic Ulcers:** Peptic ulcers are open sores on the stomach, small intestine, or esophagus lining caused by stomach acid. Common reasons include Helicobacter pylori bacteria infection, long-term use of nonsteroidal anti-inflammatory medicines (NSAIDs), and heavy alcohol use.

• **Irritable Bowel Syndrome (IBS):** IBS is a functional gastrointestinal condition marked by abdominal pain, bloating, gas, and changes in bowel habits, such as diarrhea, constipation, or both. The specific etiology of IBS is unknown, but it could be due to anomalies in the gut-brain axis, altered gut motility, or food sensitivity.

• **Inflammatory Bowel Disease (IBD):** IBD refers to two conditions: Crohn's disease and ulcerative colitis. These are chronic inflammatory illnesses of the digestive tract that cause inflammation, ulcers, and tissue destruction. The symptoms are abdominal pain, diarrhea, rectal bleeding, exhaustion, and weight loss.

• **Celiac Disease:** Celiac disease is an autoimmune illness caused by the consumption of gluten, a protein found in wheat, rye, and barley. Gluten stimulates an immunological reaction in people with celiac disease, causing damage to the lining of the small intestine and nutrient loss. Symptoms include diarrhea, stomach pain, bloating, lethargy, and weight loss.

• **Gallstones:** Gallstones are hardened deposits that develop in the gallbladder, a tiny organ that holds bile produced by the liver. Gallstones can obstruct the passage of bile and induce inflammation, resulting in symptoms such as stomach pain, nausea, vomiting, and yellowing.

• **Diverticulitis:** Diverticulitis is the inflammation or infection of tiny pouches (diverticula) that can form in the walls of the colon. It is frequently connected with a low-fiber diet and can result in symptoms such as abdominal pain, fever, nausea, and stool abnormalities.

Understanding the underlying causes, symptoms, and treatment choices for digestive diseases is critical for effective management and improved quality of life. Treatment may include dietary adjustments, medication, lifestyle changes, and, in certain situations, surgical intervention. Seeking prompt medical attention and collaborating closely with healthcare providers can assist those suffering from digestive issues to achieve better outcomes and symptom management.

Common Digestive Disorders.

Digestive diseases are common conditions affecting millions of individuals worldwide, causing discomfort, suffering, and disturbance in daily life. Below are some of the most common digestive disorders:

• **Gastroesophageal Reflux Disease (GERD):** GERD happens when stomach acid runs back into the esophagus, causing symptoms like heartburn, regurgitation, chest pain, and difficulty swallowing.

Chronic GERD can lead to complications such as esophagitis, strictures, and Barrett's esophagus.

• **Irritable Bowel Syndrome (IBS):** IBS is a functional gastrointestinal condition marked by abdominal pain, bloating, gas, and changes in bowel habits, such as diarrhea, constipation, or both. While the specific reason is uncertain, dietary changes, stress, and altered gastrointestinal motility may all contribute to symptoms.

• **Peptic Ulcers:** Peptic ulcers are open sores on the stomach, small intestine, or esophagus lining caused by Helicobacter pylori bacterium infection, long-term NSAID usage, or heavy alcohol intake. The symptoms are stomach pain, bloating, nausea, and vomiting.

• **Inflammatory Bowel Disease (IBD):** IBD refers to two conditions: Crohn's disease and ulcerative colitis. These are chronic inflammatory illnesses of the digestive tract that cause inflammation, ulcers, and tissue destruction. The symptoms are abdominal pain, diarrhea, rectal bleeding, exhaustion, and weight loss.

• **Gallstones:** Gallstones are hardened deposits that form in the gallbladder, usually as a result of bile composition imbalance. They can obstruct the passage of bile, resulting in symptoms including abdominal pain (particularly after eating fatty foods), nausea, vomiting, and jaundice.

• **Celiac Disease:** Celiac disease is an autoimmune illness caused by gluten intake, resulting in damage to the lining of the small intestine. Symptoms include diarrhea, stomach pain, bloating, lethargy, and weight loss. The treatment entails a rigorous gluten-free diet.

• **Diverticulitis:** Diverticulitis develops when pouches (diverticula) form in the walls of the colon and become inflamed or infected. Symptoms include abdominal pain (typically on the lower left side), fever, nausea, vomiting, and changes in bowel patterns. A high-fiber diet and antibiotics are popular therapies.

• **Gastroenteritis:** Gastroenteritis, often known as the stomach flu, is an inflammation of the stomach and intestines that is typically caused by viral or bacterial infections. The symptoms are diarrhea, stomach pain, nausea, vomiting, fever, and dehydration.

These are only a few examples of typical digestive issues. While some may recover with simple lifestyle modifications or medication, others necessitate continuous management and medical intervention. It is critical to contact a healthcare professional for an accurate diagnosis and therapy customized to your specific needs.

Chronic Conditions and Management

Chronic digestive diseases may necessitate long-term care techniques to alleviate symptoms, avoid complications, and enhance overall quality of life. Here are some prevalent chronic digestive diseases and associated management strategies:

Inflammatory Bowel Disorder (IBD):

• **Medications:** Anti-inflammatory medications, immunosuppressants, biologic treatments, and steroids may be recommended to alleviate inflammation and symptoms.

• **Lifestyle changes:** Eating a low-residue diet, staying hydrated, controlling stress, and engaging in regular exercise can all help reduce flare-ups.

• **Surgery:** In severe cases or complications, such as intestinal obstructions or perforations, surgery may be required to remove the damaged intestine.

Irritable Bowel Syndrome:

• **Dietary changes:** Identifying trigger foods and adhering to a low-FODMAP diet, which limits fermentable carbohydrates, can help relieve symptoms.

• **Drugs:** Antispasmodics, laxatives, and drugs to treat diarrhea or constipation may be administered based on the symptoms.

• **Stress management:** Techniques including relaxation exercises, cognitive-behavioral therapy, and mindfulness meditation can help alleviate stress symptoms.

Gastroesophageal reflux disorder (GERD):

• **Lifestyle changes:** Avoiding trigger foods (e.g., spicy, acidic, fatty foods), eating smaller meals, staying at a healthy weight, and elevating the head of the bed can all help lessen reflux symptoms.

• **Medications:** Proton pump inhibitors (PPIs), H2-receptor antagonists, and antacids can all help reduce stomach acid production and relieve symptoms.

• **Surgery:** In severe cases or when drugs fail, surgical treatments such as fundoplication may be used to reinforce the lower esophageal sphincter and prevent reflux.

Crohn's disease and ulcerative colitis:

• **Medications:** Anti-inflammatory medications, immunosuppressants, biologic treatments, and corticosteroids may be used to reduce inflammation and alleviate symptoms.

• **Dietary changes:** Some people get relief from avoiding items that cause symptoms, such as high-fiber or lactose-containing foods.

• **Surgery:** In severe cases or problems such as bowel blockages, fistulas, or colon cancer, surgery may be required to remove diseased sections of the intestine or the entire colon.

Celiac disease:

• **Gluten-free diet:** Avoiding gluten-containing foods such as wheat, barley, rye, and their derivatives is critical for managing symptoms and avoiding long-term consequences.

• **Nutritional supplements:** Because celiac disease can create dietary deficiencies, supplementation with vitamins and minerals may be required to address them.

Managing chronic digestive disorders frequently necessitates a collaborative effort among healthcare experts, including gastroenterologists, nutritionists, and mental health specialists. Individualized treatment regimens suited to each patient's unique needs and symptoms are critical for getting optimal results and enhancing quality of life.

Chapter 3: The Importance of Nutrition in Digestive Health

Nutrition plays a significant role in digestive health since the foods we eat have a direct impact on the operation of the gastrointestinal (GI) tract, the makeup of gut microbiota, and our overall health. Here are a few essential points that emphasize the importance of nutrition in digestive health:

Digestive Enzymes and Nutrient Absorption: The digestive process begins in the mouth, where enzymes in saliva degrade carbs. In the stomach, gastric fluids containing enzymes such as pepsin and hydrochloric acid further degrade protein. Pancreatic enzymes and bile from the liver help the small intestine digest and absorb carbs, proteins, and lipids. A well-balanced diet rich in fruits, vegetables, whole grains, lean proteins, and healthy fats provides an adequate amount of enzymes and nutrients for proper digestion and absorption.

Fiber and Digestive Regularity: Dietary fiber, found in fruits, vegetables, whole grains, legumes, and nuts, is essential for digestive regularity. Fiber bulks up stool softens it, and aids in the movement of waste through the digestive tract, reducing constipation and improving bowel regularity. Furthermore, certain forms of fiber, such as soluble fiber, can ferment in the colon and provide fuel for beneficial gut bacteria, helping to maintain a healthy gut microbiota.

Gut Microbiota and Digestive Wellness: The gut microbiota, which includes trillions of bacteria, fungi, and other microbes, is essential for digestion, nutrient absorption, immunological function, and general health. Consuming a wide variety of fiber-rich meals, fermented foods (e.g., yogurt, kefir, kimchi), and prebiotic-rich foods (e.g., onions, garlic, and bananas) can nourish and sustain healthy gut flora. Probiotic supplements and foods containing live beneficial bacteria may also help to keep your gut healthy.

Hydration and Digestive Function: Staying hydrated is vital for good digestive health. Water helps dissolve nutrients, moves food through the GI system, and softens feces to prevent constipation. Drinking enough water throughout the day, as well as hydrating foods like fruits and vegetables, promotes good digestive function and general health.

Identifying Trigger Foods: Identifying and avoiding trigger foods is critical for managing symptoms in people with digestive problems including irritable bowel syndrome (IBS) or food intolerances. FODMAPs, spicy foods, fatty foods, coffee, alcohol, and artificial sweeteners are all common triggers. Working with a healthcare physician or a nutritionist to create a tailored nutrition plan can help people identify trigger foods and make dietary changes to relieve symptoms and improve their quality of life.

Overall, eating a well-balanced and varied diet rich in fiber, probiotics, and hydrating fluids is essential for supporting digestive health, increasing regularity, and lowering the risk of digestive diseases. Maintaining a healthy lifestyle that includes regular physical activity, stress management, and appropriate sleep also helps to improve overall digestive health.

The Digestive process

The digestive process is a complex series of actions that begins when food enters the mouth and concludes with nutrient absorption and waste disposal. Here is a summary of the digestive process:

• **Ingestion:** The process of digestion begins with ingestion, which involves taking food into the mouth and chewing it into smaller pieces, breaking it down mechanically.

• **Salivation:** As food is digested, salivary glands in the mouth produce saliva, which contains enzymes like amylase that begin to break down carbohydrates into simpler sugars.

• **Swallowing:** After chewing and mixing with saliva, the food is shaped into a bolus and swallowed, passing down the throat (pharynx) and into the esophagus.

• **Peristalsis:** The esophagus uses repetitive muscle contractions known as peristalsis to drive the food bolus downward into the stomach.

• **Stomach:** When food enters the stomach, it is combined with gastric juices, which include hydrochloric acid and enzymes like pepsin. These acidic conditions help to break down proteins into smaller peptides and amino acids. The stomach also serves as a temporary storage reservoir for food, gradually releasing it into the small intestine.

• **Small Intestine:** The small intestine, which is separated into three sections—the duodenum, jejunum, and ileum—is where the majority of digestion and nutritional absorption takes place. Enzymes from the pancreas (e.g., pancreatic amylase, lipase, proteases) and bile from the liver (stored in the gallbladder) help break down carbs, lipids, and proteins into their constituent units. Sugars, amino acids, fatty acids, vitamins, and minerals are absorbed via the small intestine walls and into the bloodstream.

• **Large Intestine (Colon):** Any undigested food particles and waste products not absorbed in the small intestine move into the large intestine, where water and electrolytes are absorbed, resulting in feces. The colon also contains a large colony of helpful bacteria known as gut microbiota, which ferment undigested carbohydrates and create vitamins (such as vitamin K and biotin) and short-chain fatty acids.

• **Rectum and Anus:** Feces are kept in the rectum and released from the body via the anus during defecation.

Throughout the digestive process, a complex interaction of hormones, neurons, and feedback systems regulates digestive juice secretion, food transit through the GI tract, and nutrient absorption. This concerted effort ensures that vital nutrients are taken from meals, waste is properly removed, and the body receives the energy and building blocks it needs for growth, repair, and maintenance.

Nutrition and Digestive Health

Nutrients are essential for digestive health because they support gastrointestinal tract function, promote the growth of healthy gut flora, and help avoid digestive problems. Here are several crucial nutrients and their effects on digestive health:

• **Fiber:** Dietary fiber is crucial for digestive regularity and colon health. Soluble fiber, found in foods like oats, beans, and fruits, creates a gel-like substance in the digestive tract, softening stool and regulating bowel motions. Whole grains, veggies, and nuts include insoluble fiber, which bulks up the stool and promotes intestinal regularity. Furthermore, fiber acts as a prebiotic, feeding beneficial gut bacteria and promoting a healthy gut microbiota.

• **Probiotics:** Probiotics are live beneficial bacteria that can provide health advantages when ingested in sufficient quantities. These friendly microbes contribute to a healthy gut bacteria balance, immunological function, and nutritional digestion and absorption. Yogurt, kefir, sauerkraut, kimchi, and kombucha are all probiotic foods. Probiotic pills may also be good for people who have digestive issues or are taking antibiotics, which can alter the gut microbiota.

• **Digestive Enzymes:** Enzymes are proteins that help the body perform chemical reactions, such as breaking down food molecules during digestion. The salivary glands, stomach, pancreas, and small intestine all create digestive enzymes, which help break down carbs, proteins, and lipids into smaller molecules that the body can absorb and use. The creation and activation of digestive enzymes requires an adequate intake of key elements such as vitamins and minerals.

• **Water:** Staying hydrated is vital for good gut health and avoiding constipation. Water helps to dissolve nutrients, move food through the digestive tract, and soften stool, making it easier to pass. Drinking enough water throughout the day, as well as eating hydrating fruits and vegetables, promotes healthy digestion and general well-being.

• **Antioxidants:** Vitamins A, C, and E, as well as selenium, help protect digestive tract cells from damage caused by free radicals and oxidative stress. Consuming antioxidant-rich foods such as fruits, vegetables, nuts, seeds, and whole grains can help preserve digestive mucosal health and lower the risk of illnesses such as inflammatory bowel disease (IBD) and colon cancer.

• **Omega-3 Fatty Acids:** Omega-3 fatty acids, which can be found in fatty fish (such as salmon, mackerel, and sardines), flaxseeds, chia seeds, and walnuts, have anti-inflammatory properties that may help reduce inflammation in the digestive tract and alleviate symptoms of Crohn's disease, ulcerative colitis, and irritable bowel syndrome (IBS).

Overall, a well-balanced diet high in fiber, probiotics, digestive enzymes, antioxidants, and important nutrients is critical for boosting digestive health, maintaining a healthy gut flora, and lowering the risk of digestive problems. Including a variety of nutrient-dense foods in your diet and staying hydrated are essential for sustaining healthy digestive function and overall health.

Chapter 4: Gut microbiota: The Key to Digestive Wellness

Gut microbiota, also known as the gut microbiome, is a varied community of trillions of bacteria, fungi, viruses, and other microorganisms that live in the digestive tract, particularly the large intestine (colon). These microbes are essential for digestive health and overall well-being. Here's why the gut microbiota is regarded as the key to digestive health:

• **Digestive Function:** Gut microbes help break down and ferment dietary fibers and other complex carbohydrates that humans cannot digest on their own. During this process, they produce short-chain fatty acids (SCFAs) such as acetate, propionate, and butyrate, which serve as an energy source for colon cells and aid in the maintenance of the intestinal barrier. Gut bacteria also create enzymes and metabolites that help in nutrition digestion and absorption.

• **Immune Regulation:** The gut microbiota regulates immune function and protects against infections. Beneficial bacteria help the immune system learn to distinguish between hazardous invaders and safe antigens, lowering the risk of inflammatory and autoimmune reactions. They also produce antibiotic chemicals and compete with pathogenic bacteria for nutrition and colonization sites, thereby promoting a healthy microbial community.

• **Metabolic Health:** A new study indicates that the makeup and variety of the gut microbiota influence metabolic processes such as energy metabolism, lipid metabolism, and glucose homeostasis. Imbalances in the gut microbiome, defined as a decrease in beneficial bacteria and an increase in harmful bacteria, have been linked to illnesses such as obesity, type 2 diabetes, and metabolic syndrome. In contrast, promoting a healthy gut microbiome through dietary changes and probiotic supplements may benefit metabolic health and weight management.

• **Brain-Gut Axis:** The brain-gut axis is a network of neurological, hormonal, and immunological processes that connects the gut microbiota to the central nervous system in both directions. This communication system is critical for regulating mood, cognition, and behavior, and it has been linked to the development of mental health problems like as anxiety, depression, and stress-related illnesses. Certain gut bacteria create neurotransmitters and neuroactive chemicals that affect brain function, whilst others regulate the synthesis of stress hormones and inflammatory cytokines.

• **Digestive Disorders:** Dysbiosis, or imbalances in the gut microbiota, has been related to the development and worsening of a variety of digestive ailments, including irritable bowel syndrome (IBS), inflammatory bowel disease (IBD), gastroesophageal reflux disease (GERD), and celiac disease. Restoring microbial balance by dietary changes, probiotic supplementation, and fecal microbiota transplantation (FMT) shows promise as a treatment strategy for controlling these disorders and improving digestive health.

To summarize, the gut microbiota contributes to digestive health, immunological function, metabolic health, and brain-gut communication. Supporting a diverse and balanced gut microbiota through a fiber-rich diet, fermented foods, and prebiotics, as well as lifestyle variables such as regular exercise, stress management, and appropriate sleep, is critical for supporting overall digestive health and well-being.

The Gut Microbiome: Fundamentals and Importance

The gut microbiome is the diverse collection of bacteria that live in the gastrointestinal tract, particularly the large intestine (colon). The gut microbiome, which contains trillions of bacteria, fungi, viruses, and other microorganisms, plays an important role in human health and well-being. Here is an overview of the gut microbiota and its significance:

• **Diversity:** The gut microbiome contains thousands of different types of bacteria and other microbes. Every person has a distinct microbiome that is influenced by genetics, nutrition, environment, age, and lifestyle.

• **Composition:** Bacterial phyla that dominate the gut microbiome are Firmicutes, Bacteroidetes, Actinobacteria, Proteobacteria, and Verrucomicrobia.

These bacteria perform a variety of tasks, including digesting dietary fibers, generating vitamins (such as B vitamins and vitamin K), metabolizing bile acids, and influencing immunological responses.

• **Function:** The gut microbiota provides critical tasks for human health, including:

• **Digestion and metabolism:** Gut bacteria help to break down food fibers, carbs, and other complex compounds, resulting in the production of short-chain fatty acids (SCFAs) and other metabolites that serve as energy and signaling molecules.

• **Immune modulation:** Gut microbiota communicate with the immune system, educating and regulating immune responses. Beneficial bacteria increase immunological tolerance and defend against infections, but dysbiosis (microbial imbalance) can lead to inflammatory and autoimmune diseases.

• **Nutrient synthesis:** Certain gut bacteria create vitamins (e.g., vitamin K and biotin) and other bioactive chemicals required for human health.

• **Barrier function:** Gut microbiota contribute to the integrity of the intestinal barrier, preventing dangerous infections and poisons from crossing into the bloodstream.

• **Importance:** The gut microbiota is becoming recognized as a critical factor of general health and disease. It plays an important function in

• **Digestive health:** A healthy gut microbiome promotes proper digestion, nutritional absorption, and bowel regularity, whereas dysbiosis is linked to digestive illnesses such as irritable bowel syndrome (IBS), inflammatory bowel disease (IBD), and gastroesophageal reflux disease (GERD).

• **Immunological function:** Gut bacteria affect immunological development, modulation, and responsiveness. Immune tolerance and pathogen resistance require a broad and balanced gut microbiota.

• **Metabolic health:** New research indicates that the gut microbiota regulates metabolism, energy control, and susceptibility to metabolic illnesses like obesity, type 2 diabetes, and cardiovascular disease.

• **Brain-gut communication:** The gut microbiome communicates bidirectionally with the central nervous system via the gut-brain axis, which influences mood, cognition, behavior, and stress responses. Anxiety, sadness, and autism spectrum disorders have all been linked to altered gut flora.

In general, the gut microbiome has a significant impact on human health and disease, influencing different physiological systems and contributing to general well-being. Maintaining a diverse and balanced gut microbiome through dietary and lifestyle changes is critical for improving digestive health, immunological function, metabolic health, and mental well-being.

Cultivating a healthy gut microbiome.

Cultivating a healthy gut microbiota is critical for improving digestive health, immunological function, metabolic health, and general well-being. Here are some techniques for promoting a diverse and balanced gut microbiome:

• **Dietary Fiber:** Eating a fiber-rich diet is one of the most effective methods to maintain a healthy gut flora. Fiber acts as a prebiotic, feeding healthy gut bacteria and increasing microbial diversity. To improve your fiber intake, eat plenty of fruits and vegetables, whole grains, legumes, nuts, and seeds.

• **Fermented Foods:** Add fermented foods to your diet to promote helpful probiotic microorganisms. Yogurt, kefir, sauerkraut, kimchi, miso, tempeh, and kombucha are some examples. These foods include live cultures of beneficial bacteria that can colonize the gut and promote microbial diversity.

• **Prebiotic Foods:** Prebiotics are non-digestible fibers that provide energy for good gut flora. Include prebiotic-rich foods in your diet, such as onions, garlic, leeks, asparagus, bananas, apples, oats, and flaxseeds, to help healthy bacteria develop in the stomach.

• **Limit Sugar and Processed Foods:** Consuming too much sugar and processed foods can upset the balance of gut bacteria and encourage the growth of harmful germs. Limit your intake of sugary snacks, desserts, sugary drinks, refined grains, and processed meals, as these can all contribute to gut dysbiosis and inflammation.

• **Probiotic Supplements:** Consider taking probiotic supplements that contain healthy bacteria types such as Lactobacillus and Bifidobacterium. To maintain gut health, take a high-quality probiotic supplement that contains a variety of bacterial strains and colony-forming units (CFUs).

• **Avoid Antibiotics When Not Necessary:** Antibiotics can upset the balance of gut flora by killing both dangerous and beneficial germs. Avoid needless antibiotic use and consult your healthcare practitioner about other treatment choices. If you must take antibiotics, try taking probiotics to promote gut health during and after treatment.

• **Stress Management:** Chronic stress can harm the gut microbiome and impair digestive function. To promote a healthy gut-brain connection, use stress-reduction practices such as mindfulness meditation, deep breathing exercises, yoga, tai chi, or spending time in nature.

• **Regular Exercise:** Physical activity has been found to improve the composition and variety of the gut microbiota. To enhance general health and a healthy gut flora, engage in regular exercise, such as aerobic activities, weight training, and flexibility exercises.

• **Adequate Sleep:** Prioritize quality sleep, since insufficient sleep can affect circadian cycles and harm gut health. Aim for 7-9 hours of undisturbed sleep per night to help the gut-brain axis work properly and improve overall health.

• **Hydration:** Drink plenty of water throughout the day to promote digestive health and stay hydrated. Hydration is necessary for moving food through the digestive tract, avoiding constipation, and enhancing nutritional absorption.

By implementing these practices into your daily routine, you can help cultivate a healthy gut flora and promote digestive well-being. Remember that individual responses to dietary and lifestyle interventions may differ, so listen to your body and make modifications depending on your specific requirements and preferences.

Chapter 5: Lifestyle Factors and Digestive Health.

Lifestyle choices have an important part in maintaining digestive health and preventing digestive problems. Here are some important lifestyle behaviors that help improve intestinal wellness:

• **Healthy Diet:** A well-balanced and diverse diet rich in fruits, vegetables, whole grains, lean meats, and healthy fats provides the nutrients and fiber required for proper digestive function. Consuming fewer processed foods, sugary snacks, and saturated fats might help prevent digestive problems like constipation, indigestion, and heartburn.

• **Hydration:** Proper hydration is necessary for digestive health. Drinking enough water throughout the day softens stool, prevents constipation, and aids in the passage of food through the digestive system. Drink at least 8-10 glasses of water every day and consume water-rich foods such as fruits and vegetables.

• **Regular Physical Activity:** Regular exercise benefits overall health and can improve digestive function. Physical activity promotes bowel movements, increases intestinal transit time, and lowers the risk of constipation and bloating. Aim for no less than 30 minutes of moderate-intensity exercise on most days of the week.

• **Stress Management:** Chronic stress can harm digestive health by changing gut flora balance, causing inflammation, and intensifying symptoms of digestive diseases such as irritable bowel syndrome (IBS). To encourage calm and a healthy gut-brain connection, try stress-reduction practices like mindfulness meditation, deep breathing exercises, yoga, or spending time outside.

• **Consistent Meal Timing:** Sticking to normal meal times and eating habits will help regulate digestive function and prevent symptoms like indigestion, bloating, and reflux. Aim to eat balanced meals at consistent times throughout the day and avoid missing meals or eating large meals late at night, which can upset digestion.

• **Avoiding Smoking and Excessive Alcohol:** Both smoking and excessive alcohol intake can hurt digestive health. Smoking raises the risk of gastrointestinal problems such as peptic ulcers, GERD, and colorectal cancer, whereas alcohol can irritate the digestive system, disturb gut bacteria, and worsen conditions including gastritis and liver disease. Quit smoking and restrict alcohol use to improve intestinal health.

• **Adequate Sleep:** Get enough restful sleep every night, as insufficient sleep can disrupt digestive function and aggravate symptoms of digestive illnesses such as IBS and GERD. Aim for 7-9 hours of excellent sleep per night, and create a soothing bedtime routine to promote good sleep habits.

• **Maintaining a Healthy Weight:** Obesity and excess weight might raise the risk of digestive problems such as GERD, gallstones, fatty liver disease, and colon cancer. A healthy lifestyle that includes a balanced diet, regular exercise, and stress management will help you maintain a healthy weight and improve digestive health.

By adopting these lifestyle elements into your everyday routine, you can enhance digestive health, lower your risk of digestive problems, and general well-being. It is critical to listen to your body, pay attention to digestive symptoms, and seek medical assistance if you have persistent or severe digestive problems.

Stress Management Techniques

Managing stress is critical for general well-being, including digestion. Here are some excellent stress management practices that might aid in relaxation and digestive wellness:

• **Mindfulness Meditation:** In mindfulness meditation, you focus your attention on the present moment without judgment. Regular mindfulness meditation can help reduce stress, anxiety, and rumination, resulting in increased emotional well-being and digestion.

• **Deep Breathing Exercises:** Deep breathing exercises, such as diaphragmatic breathing or belly breathing, can trigger the body's relaxation response and assist in calming the nervous system. Take slow, deep breaths to fill your abdomen with oxygen, then slowly exhale through your mouth. Repeat this method multiple times to help you relax and lessen stress.

• **Progressive Muscle Relaxation (PMR):** In PMR, different muscle groups in the body are gradually tensed and subsequently relaxed. By intentionally relaxing stiff muscles, you can relieve physical tension and produce a sense of relaxation throughout your body, which can help with stress relief and digestion.

• **Yoga:** Yoga is a combination of physical postures, breathing exercises, and meditation that promotes relaxation, flexibility, and stress reduction. Regular yoga practice can help lower cortisol levels (the stress hormone) and improve digestion by relaxing the nervous system and encouraging mindful eating habits.

• **Tai Chi:** Tai Chi is a calm mind-body exercise that combines slow, flowing motions with deep breathing.

Regular Tai Chi practice can help reduce stress, anxiety, and muscle tension while also encouraging relaxation and overall well-being, including digestive health.

• **Nature Walks:** Spending time in nature can have a relaxing impact on the mind and body, lowering tension and increasing relaxation. Take leisurely walks in natural settings like parks, forests, or beaches to reconnect with nature, clear your thoughts, and revitalize your spirit.

• **Journaling:** Recording your thoughts, feelings, and experiences in a journal can help you achieve clarity, process emotions, and reduce stress. Spend a few minutes each day journaling about your thoughts and emotions, with a focus on thankfulness, happy experiences, and stress-reduction strategies.

• **Social Support:** Connecting with friends, family, or support groups can provide emotional support while also mitigating the consequences of stress. Share your emotions with trustworthy loved ones, seek advice or encouragement, and participate in important social activities to boost your sense of belonging and reduce stress.

• **Hobbies and Creative Activities:** Engaging in enjoyable hobbies and creative activities can assist in diverting your attention away from pressures and encourage relaxation. Whether it's painting, gardening, music, or cooking, choose hobbies that make you happy and allow you to express yourself artistically.

• **Limiting Screen Time:** Excessive screen time, particularly on electronic devices such as cellphones, computers, and televisions, can cause stress and alter sleep patterns. Set screen time limits, take breaks from electronic devices, and participate in soothing activities that encourage mindfulness and stress alleviation.

Incorporating these stress management practices into your daily routine can assist to reduce tension, increase relaxation, and improve digestive health. Experiment with different strategies to see what works best for you, and prioritize self-care to ensure overall well-being.

Exercise and Its Effect on Digestion

Exercise promotes digestive health and supports optimal digestion. Here's how exercise affects digestion.

• **Increased Bowel Regularity:** Regular physical activity, such as aerobic exercise, walking, or running, can stimulate bowel motions and increase bowel regularity. Exercise activates gastrointestinal muscles, allowing food to pass more easily through the digestive system and lowering the risk of constipation.

• **Reduced Risk of Digestive Disorders:** Regular exercise has been linked to a lower risk of constipation, irritable bowel syndrome (IBS), inflammatory bowel disease (IBD), and gastroesophageal reflux disease (GERD). Exercise improves bowel function, reduces inflammation, and promotes overall digestive health.

• **Weight Management:** Regular exercise will help you maintain a healthy weight and avoid obesity, which is a risk factor for digestive illnesses like GERD, gallstones, fatty liver disease, and colon cancer. Exercise enhances energy expenditure, metabolism, and appropriate weight control, all of which improve digestive health.

• **Stress Reduction:** Exercise is a powerful stress-reduction approach that can help lower stress levels and improve relaxation. Chronic stress can impair digestion by affecting gut motility, causing inflammation, and intensifying symptoms of digestive diseases such as IBS and GERD. Regular exercise regulates stress hormones like cortisol and fosters a healthy gut-brain link.

• **Increased Gut Motility:** Exercise activates the muscles of the gastrointestinal tract, boosting gut motility and assisting in the movement of food through the digestive system. Physical activity promotes regular bowel movements, which aids digestion and lowers the risk of diseases such as constipation and bloating.

• **Increased Blood Flow to Digestive Organs:** Exercise boosts blood flow to the digestive organs, such as the stomach, intestines, and colon, which improves nutrition delivery, promotes tissue repair, and promotes normal digestive function. Improved blood flow can help prevent ischemic colitis and improve overall gastrointestinal health.

• **Support for Gut Microbiome:** New research indicates that regular exercise can improve the composition and diversity of gut microbiota, the beneficial bacteria that live in the digestive tract. Exercise may help establish a healthy gut flora, lower inflammation, and boost immune function, all of which are necessary for digestive health.

• **Reduced Digestive Disorder Symptoms:** Exercise can help with the symptoms of some digestive disorders, such as IBS and functional dyspepsia. While intense exercise can worsen symptoms in some people with digestive disorders, moderate-intensity exercise has been shown to improve symptoms and quality of life in many cases.

To summarize, regular exercise promotes digestive health and overall well-being. By encouraging bowel regularity, reducing stress, supporting weight management, enhancing gut motility, and improving blood supply to the digestive organs, exercise contributes to good digestion and reduces the risk of digestive problems. Incorporate a combination of aerobic exercise, strength training, flexibility exercises, and relaxation techniques into your routine to support gut wellness and preserve overall health.

Chapter 6: Digestive Health Across Life Stages

Digestive health is important at all stages of life, from infancy to old age. Here's a quick rundown of gut health factors and guidelines for various life stages:

Infant and Early Childhood:

• Breastfeeding: Breast milk contains critical nutrients and antibodies that help babies establish a healthy digestive and immunological system. Exclusive breastfeeding is suggested for the first six months of life, followed by continuing breastfeeding and the introduction of complementary foods.

• **Introduction of Solid Foods:** Introducing a range of nutrient-dense, age-appropriate solid foods during infancy and early childhood promotes healthy growth and development. Gradually introduce new foods to detect any sensitivities or intolerances and promote good eating habits.

Childhood & Adolescence:

• **Balanced Diet:** Encourage children and adolescents to eat fruits, vegetables, whole grains, lean proteins, and healthy fats. Limit your intake of sugary snacks, processed foods, and sugary beverages, as these might have a bad impact on your digestive health and overall well-being.

• **Hydration:** Encourage kids to drink plenty of water all day. Limit your use of sugary and caffeinated beverages, which can lead to dehydration and stomach problems.

Adulthood:

• **Healthy Eating Habits:** Eat a balanced diet and practice healthy eating habits to improve digestive health and general well-being. Include fiber-rich foods, probiotics, and prebiotics in your diet to improve gut health and prevent digestive problems.

• **Regular Physical exercise:** Regular physical exercise promotes bowel regularity, reduces stress, and supports optimum digestion. To maintain general health, combine aerobic activity with strength training and flexibility activities.

• **Regular Health Screenings:** Schedule regular check-ups with your doctor to monitor your digestive health and screen for illnesses like colorectal cancer, irritable bowel syndrome (IBS), and gastroesophageal reflux disease (GERD). Follow the suggested screening standards based on age, family history, and risk factors.

Older adults:

• **Nutrient Absorption:** As we age, our bodies' ability to absorb certain nutrients declines. Consume nutrient-dense foods and, if necessary, take supplements to support optimal nutrient absorption and digestive function.

• **Hydration:** Because of changes in thirst perception and renal function with age, older persons may be more susceptible to dehydration. Drink plenty of water and eat hydrating meals like fruits and vegetables to stay hydrated and promote digestive health.

• **Medication Management:** Older persons may be more prone to take digestive-related drugs, such as proton pump inhibitors (PPIs), laxatives, and painkillers. Collaborate with healthcare experts to control drugs and reduce potential side effects on digestive function.

Throughout life, it is critical to pay attention to digestive symptoms, seek medical guidance if they continue or are troubling, and make lifestyle choices that promote optimal digestive health. Individuals can enhance gut wellness and improve their quality of life at any time by eating healthily, staying hydrated, engaging in regular physical activity, and getting appropriate medical care.

Digestive health between infancy and childhood

Digestive health during infancy and children is critical to growth, development, and overall well-being. Here are a few key items to consider.

• **Breastfeeding:** Breastfeeding is the gold standard for newborn nutrition and plays an important role in digestive health. Breast milk provides vital nutrients, antibodies, and good bacteria that contribute to healthy gut microbiota, defend against infections and promote appropriate digestion and nutrient absorption.

• **Introduction of Solid Foods:** Solid foods are normally introduced at about 6 months of age. Introduce a range of age-appropriate, nutrient-dense foods to promote healthy growth and development. Gradually introduce new foods to check for allergies or intolerances, and encourage healthy eating habits from a young age.

• **Fiber and Hydration:** As children go to solid foods, they must ingest an adequate amount of dietary fiber and remain hydrated. Fiber-rich meals like fruits, vegetables, whole grains, and legumes improve digestive health by promoting bowel regularity and avoiding constipation. Encourage youngsters to drink water throughout the day to stay hydrated and promote appropriate digestion.

• **Probiotics and prebiotics:** Probiotics are beneficial bacteria that promote digestive health by balancing the gut flora. Prebiotics are non-digestible fibers that act as food for probiotics, allowing them to thrive in the gut. Consuming probiotic-rich foods like yogurt, kefir, and fermented foods, as well as prebiotic-rich foods like bananas, onions, and whole grains, can help infants develop a healthy gut flora.

• **Healthy Eating Habits:** Promote healthy eating habits in children by providing a range of nutritious foods and demonstrating positive eating behaviors. Limit your intake of sugary snacks, processed foods, and sugary beverages, as these might have a bad impact on your digestive health and overall well-being.

• **Physical Activity:** Regular physical activity is beneficial for children's general health, including digestive health. Encourage vigorous play, sports, and outdoor activities to increase bowel regularity, reduce stress, and improve overall health.

• **Routine Healthcare Visits:** Schedule routine healthcare checkups, such as well-child check-ups and immunizations. Discuss any concerns you have about your child's digestive issues, growth, or development with their doctor, and follow suggested screening recommendations for disorders including celiac disease, food allergies, and lactose intolerance.

• **Food Allergies and Intolerances:** Be aware of any potential food allergies or intolerances in children, and take steps to detect and manage them. Common dietary allergies include cow's milk, eggs, peanuts, tree nuts, soy, wheat, fish, and shellfish. If you suspect your child has a food allergy or intolerance, check with a healthcare expert for accurate diagnosis and treatment.

Parents and caregivers can support optimal digestive health in infancy and childhood by focusing on breastfeeding, introducing nutritious foods, supporting water and fiber consumption, encouraging physical exercise, and addressing any concerns about food allergies or intolerances. Regular medical checkups and open contact with healthcare providers are critical for tracking growth, development, and overall well-being throughout childhood.

Digestive Changes between Adolescence and Adulthood.

Several changes occur in the digestive system between adolescence and adulthood that might have an impact on digestive health and overall well-being. Here are some typical digestive changes and considerations during different life stages:

• **Puberty and hormone Changes:** Adolescent hormone changes, such as increases in estrogen and testosterone, can have an impact on digestive function. These hormonal oscillations may have an impact on gastrointestinal motility, stomach acid secretion, and hunger modulation, potentially resulting in symptoms including bloating, abdominal discomfort, and changes in bowel habits. A balanced diet, frequent physical activity, and stress management practices can all assist promote gut health during this transitional phase.

• **Dietary Habits and Lifestyle Factors:** As people enter adulthood, their eating habits and lifestyle choices can have a substantial impact on their digestive health. Busy schedules, increased stress levels, and changes in eating habits can all lead to poor dietary choices, irregular meal times, and overconsumption of processed foods, all of which can disrupt digestive function and contribute to gastrointestinal problems like indigestion, heartburn, and constipation. A balanced diet rich in fruits, vegetables, whole grains, lean proteins, and healthy fats, as well as regular physical activity and stress management, can help maintain good digestive health in adulthood.

• **Stress and Digestive Function:** Stress is a major cause of digestive problems at any age. Academic difficulties, employment responsibilities, marital issues, and other life stressors can all contribute to increased stress during youth and adulthood. Chronic stress can affect gut microbial balance, alter gastrointestinal motility, and worsen symptoms of digestive diseases such as irritable bowel syndrome (IBS) and functional dyspepsia. Stress-reduction practices such as mindfulness meditation, deep breathing exercises, yoga, and regular physical activity can all aid in relaxation and digestive health.

• **Digestive Disorders and Chronic Conditions:** Adolescents and adults may be more likely to develop digestive disorders and chronic conditions like gastroesophageal reflux disease (GERD), irritable bowel syndrome (IBS), inflammatory bowel disease (IBD), celiac disease, and food intolerances. These diseases can result in stomach pain, bloating, diarrhea, constipation, and gastrointestinal discomfort. Seeking medical examination and treatment from a healthcare provider is critical for managing symptoms, determining underlying reasons, and enhancing digestive health.

• **Medication Use:** As people get older, they may be more prone to take drugs that impact digestive function. Common medications, such as nonsteroidal anti-inflammatory drugs (NSAIDs), proton pump inhibitors (PPIs), antibiotics, and certain prescription medications, can disrupt gut microbiota balance, increase the risk of gastrointestinal bleeding or ulcers, or cause symptoms like diarrhea and constipation. It is critical to take drugs as prescribed by a healthcare provider and to discuss any potential side effects or concerns about digestive health.

Adolescents and adults can support optimal digestive health and general well-being throughout their lives by adopting good lifestyle behaviors, managing stress, seeking medical examinations for digestive problems, and making informed drug usage decisions. Regular healthcare visits and open communication with healthcare practitioners are critical for assessing digestive function, treating issues, and promoting long-term digestive health.

Aging and Digestive Wellness

As people age, their digestive systems undergo a variety of changes that might have an impact on their overall health. Here are some typical age-related changes and concerns for supporting digestive health in older adults:

• **Decreased Digestive Enzyme Production:** As we age, the body's ability to produce digestive enzymes including lactase, lipase, and stomach acid decreases. This can cause less food absorption, delayed digestion, and an increased risk of vitamin shortages. To aid digestion, older persons may benefit from eating smaller, more often meals, selecting easily digestible foods, and taking digestive enzyme supplements if advised by a healthcare provider.

• **Reduced Gastric Motility:** As we age, our gastric motility declines, resulting in delayed stomach emptying and an increased risk of gastrointestinal symptoms like bloating, indigestion, and reflux. Eating fewer meals, avoiding large or heavy meals late in the day, and standing upright after eating can all help alleviate stomach reflux symptoms and improve digestion.

• **Changes in Gut Microbiota:** Aging is connected with changes in the composition and diversity of gut microbiota, which are beneficial bacteria that live in the digestive tract. These changes may have an impact on immunological function, nutrient absorption, and gastrointestinal health. A healthy gut microbiome can be supported by older persons eating a diet high in fiber, probiotics, and prebiotics, as well as engaging in regular physical activity and stress management.

• **Constipation and Bowel Disorders:** Constipation is a common digestive complaint in older adults, which is frequently attributed to causes such as decreased physical activity, dietary changes, medication use, and age-related changes in bowel function. To avoid and treat constipation, older persons should eat a fiber-rich diet, stay hydrated, engage in regular physical exercise, and practice good bowel habits. In some circumstances, laxatives or stool softeners may be prescribed by a healthcare provider.

• **Medication Use:** Older persons are more likely to use several medications, which can impair digestive function and raise the risk of gastrointestinal complications such as nausea, diarrhea, constipation, and gastrointestinal bleeding. Older persons should evaluate their drug regimen with their healthcare practitioner frequently, consider any interactions or adverse effects, and take medications exactly as prescribed.

• **Hydration and Fluid Intake:** Older persons may be more prone to dehydration due to age-related changes in thirst perception, renal function, and overall fluid balance. Dehydration can worsen constipation, urinary tract infections, and other medical problems. Encourage older folks to drink lots of water throughout the day, eat hydrating meals like fruits and vegetables, and limit their intake of diuretic beverages like coffee and alcohol.

• **Regular Healthcare Visits:** To monitor digestive health, address any concerns or symptoms, and receive appropriate screening tests for conditions such as colorectal cancer, gastroesophageal reflux disease (GERD), and inflammatory bowel disease (IBD), older adults should schedule regular healthcare visits with their primary care physician or gastroenterologist. Early identification and treatment of digestive diseases is critical for supporting optimal digestive health and well-being in older persons.

Addressing age-related changes in digestion, adopting good lifestyle practices, regulating medication use, staying hydrated, and obtaining regular medical treatment can help older persons maintain digestive wellness and have a greater quality of life as they age. Open communication with healthcare practitioners and proactive management of digestive symptoms are essential for maintaining excellent digestive health in later life.

Chapter 7: Diagnostic Tools and Treatment Options.

The diagnostic methods and therapy options for digestive disorders differ based on the specific ailment and its underlying cause. The following are some common diagnostic techniques and treatment strategies used in gastroenterology:

Diagnostic tools:

a. **Medical History and Physical Examination:** In many cases, identifying digestive issues begins with a complete medical history and physical examination. To guide further examination and treatment, healthcare providers consider symptoms, risk factors, and a patient's medical history.

b. **Laboratory Tests:** Blood tests, stool tests, and other laboratory testing may be used to detect abnormalities such as inflammation, infection, nutritional deficiencies, or gastrointestinal disease markers.

c. **Imaging Studies:** Imaging studies such as X-rays, ultrasounds, computed tomography (CT) scans, magnetic resonance imaging (MRI), and endoscopic ultrasound (EUS) can be used to examine the gastrointestinal tract, identify structural abnormalities, and assess disease severity.

d. **Endoscopic Procedures:** Endoscopy is putting a flexible tube with a camera (endoscope) into the digestive tract to view the esophagus, stomach, small intestine, or colon. Endoscopic procedures such as esophagogastroduodenoscopy (EGD), colonoscopy, sigmoidoscopy, and capsule endoscopy can be used to diagnose disorders, collect tissue samples (biopsies), and carry out therapeutic operations.

e. **Manometry:** Esophageal manometry monitors pressure and muscular contractions in the esophagus to assess swallowing function, esophageal motility abnormalities, and diseases including gastroesophageal reflux disease (GERD).

f. **Breath testing:** Breath testing can help detect lactose intolerance, bacterial overgrowth in the small intestine, and Helicobacter pylori infection.

Treatment Options:

a. **Medications:** Pharmacological therapies are frequently utilized to treat the symptoms and underlying diseases associated with digestive disorders. Antacids, proton pump inhibitors (PPIs), H2-receptor antagonists, antibiotics, antispasmodics, laxatives, anti-inflammatory medicines, immunosuppressants, and biologic treatments are all possible medications.

b. **Dietary Modifications:** Many digestive illnesses can be managed through dietary changes and modifications. Individuals with GERD, for example, may benefit from avoiding spicy, caffeine-containing, and acidic foods, which can aggravate symptoms. Celiac disease patients must follow a rigorous gluten-free diet, although individuals with inflammatory bowel disease (IBD) may benefit from a low-residue diet during flare-ups.

c. **Lifestyle Modifications:** Lifestyle interventions such as weight management, smoking cessation, stress reduction strategies, and dietary changes can all help manage digestive issues and promote overall health.

d. **Endoscopic and Surgical Interventions:** Certain digestive problems may require endoscopic procedures and surgical interventions to be diagnosed and treated. Examples include endoscopic mucosal resection (EMR), endoscopic submucosal dissection (ESD), polypectomy, stricture dilatation, stent implantation, and surgical resection.

e. **Nutritional Support:** People suffering from malnutrition, nutritional deficiencies, or conditions that impair nutrient absorption may require nutritional support, such as dietary counseling, nutritional supplements, enteral nutrition (tube feeding), or parenteral nutrition (intravenous feeding).

f. **Behavioral Therapy:** Cognitive-behavioral therapy (CBT) or biofeedback may be prescribed for addressing stress-related or psychologically affected ailments such as irritable bowel syndrome (IBS) or functional gastrointestinal disorders (FGIDs).

g. **Follow-Up Care:** Regular follow-up visits with a gastroenterologist or other healthcare practitioner are critical for monitoring symptoms, assessing therapy effectiveness, and changing management techniques as needed.

Overall, managing digestive issues necessitates a multidisciplinary strategy that includes healthcare providers, gastroenterologists, dietitians, psychologists, and other specialists who work together to provide complete therapy that is personalized to each patient's unique needs. Treatment approaches may include a combination of pharmaceutical medications, dietary adjustments, lifestyle changes, and procedural interventions to promote gut health and quality of life.

Diagnostic Tests for Digestive Disorders

There are different diagnostic tests available to analyze and diagnose various digestive diseases. The following are some frequent diagnostic tests used in gastroenterology:

Endoscopy:

• **Esophagogastroduodenoscopy (EGD):** This procedure entails putting a flexible tube with a camera (endoscope) via the mouth to view the esophagus, stomach, and upper part of the small intestine. EGD is used to detect disorders such as gastroesophageal reflux disease (GERD), peptic ulcers, gastritis, and Barrett's esophagus.

• **Colonoscopy:** This procedure involves putting an endoscope into the rectum to view the colon and rectum. It is used to test for colorectal cancer, detect polyps, and diagnose disorders like inflammatory bowel disease (IBD), diverticulosis, and colorectal polyps.

Imaging studies:

• **X-rays:** X-rays of the abdomen can be used to see the digestive organs and detect anomalies like intestinal obstruction, perforation, or foreign bodies.

• **Computed Tomography (CT) Scan:** CT scans produce detailed images of the belly and pelvis, which can be used to diagnose illnesses such as diverticulitis, intestinal obstruction, appendicitis, and abdominal tumors.

• **Magnetic Resonance Imaging (MRI):** MRI scans can be used to see the digestive organs and surrounding structures, as well as diagnose diseases like liver illness, pancreatic tumors, and bile duct anomalies.

• **Ultrasonography:** Abdominal ultrasonography can be used to examine the liver, gallbladder, pancreas, and bile ducts for abnormalities such as gallstones, liver cysts, or pancreatic malignancies.

Lab tests:

• **Blood Tests:** Blood tests can be used to evaluate liver function, pancreatic enzymes, inflammatory markers, and nutritional status. Common blood tests are liver function tests (LFTs), pancreatic enzyme tests (amylase and lipase), complete blood count (CBC), and C-reactive protein (CRP).

• **Stool Tests:** Stool tests can identify blood in the stool (fecal occult blood test), check for infection (stool culture), or diagnose disorders like inflammatory bowel disease (fecal calprotectin) or malabsorption (stool fat content).

Breathing Tests:

• **Hydrogen Breath Test:** This test is used to diagnose disorders like lactose intolerance, bacterial overgrowth in the small intestine, and carbohydrate malabsorption. Patients consume a certain substrate (such as lactose or glucose), and breath samples are taken to determine hydrogen levels.

Manometry:

• **Esophageal Manometry:** Esophageal manometry uses pressure and muscular contractions in the esophagus to assess swallowing function, esophageal motility problems, and conditions such as achalasia or diffuse esophageal spasm.

Biopsy:

• **Tissue Biopsy:** During an endoscopy or colonoscopy, tissue samples (biopsies) may be collected from the digestive tract for microscopic inspection. Biopsies are used to diagnose illnesses such as celiac disease, inflammatory bowel disease (IBD), Helicobacter pylori infection, and gastrointestinal cancer.

Capsule endoscopy:

• **Capsule Endoscopy:** Capsule endoscopy involves the patient swallowing a small capsule with a camera that records images of the small intestine as it travels through the digestive tract. Capsule endoscopy is used to diagnose Crohn's disease, small bowel tumors, and gastrointestinal bleeding.

These are only a few of the diagnostic tests used in gastroenterology to assess and diagnose digestive issues. The diagnostic test(s) used is determined by the patient's symptoms, medical history, and probable underlying disease. Gastroenterologists or other digestive health specialists are often responsible for interpreting test results and developing treatment plans.

Conventional and Alternative Treatment Approaches

Depending on the exact illness, degree of symptoms, and individual preferences, digestive disorders can be managed using both traditional and alternative therapeutic options. Here's a summary of traditional and alternative treatments for digestive disorders:

Conventional treatment approaches:

a. **Medications:** Pharmacological therapies are frequently used in traditional medicine to control the symptoms and underlying diseases associated with digestive disorders. Examples of drugs used to treat digestive issues are:

• Acid reflux and peptic ulcer treatments include proton pump inhibitors (PPIs) and H2-receptor antagonists.

• Antispasmodics and smooth muscle relaxants are used to treat irritable bowel syndrome.

• Antibiotics for bacterial illnesses, such as Helicobacter pylori or SIBO.

• Anti-inflammatory medications (e.g., corticosteroids, immunosuppressants) for inflammatory bowel illnesses (IBD), including Crohn's disease and ulcerative colitis.

• To treat constipation, take laxatives, stool softeners, or fiber supplements.

b. **Endoscopic and Surgical Interventions:** Endoscopic procedures or surgical interventions may be required to diagnose or treat specific digestive diseases. Examples include:

• Early-stage gastrointestinal cancers can be treated by endoscopic mucosal resection (EMR) or endoscopic submucosal dissection (ESD).

• Polypectomy is the removal of colon polyps.

• Esophageal or colon strictures can be treated with stent insertion or dilatation.

• Surgical resection for colon cancer, diverticulitis, or inflammatory bowel disease (IBD).

c. **Dietary and Lifestyle Changes:** Dietary and lifestyle changes are frequently used in conventional treatment to alleviate symptoms and improve digestive health. Examples include:

• Following a low-acid diet or avoiding foods that cause acid reflux.

• Using a low-FODMAP diet to treat irritable bowel syndrome.

• Eat smaller, more frequent meals and avoid spicy or greasy foods to treat functional dyspepsia.

• Consuming a well-balanced diet, staying hydrated, and engaging in regular physical activity help support overall digestive health.

Alternative Treatment Approaches:

a. **Nutritional treatment:** To improve digestive health, alternative medicine practitioners may use nutritional treatment, dietary supplements, and herbal therapies. Examples include:

• Probiotics and prebiotics help to maintain a healthy gut microbiome and digestive function.

• Digestive enzymes to help digest particular foods and boost nutrient absorption.

• Use herbal supplements like peppermint oil, ginger, or artichoke extract to treat indigestion, bloating, or gas.

b. **Acupuncture and Traditional Chinese Medicine (TCM):** Acupuncture and TCM can help treat digestive issues by restoring balance and boosting energy flow (Qi) throughout the body. To treat symptoms like nausea, abdominal discomfort, or diarrhea, acupuncture points connected to the digestive tract can be treated.

c. **Mind-Body Therapies:** Mindfulness meditation, yoga, and hypnotherapy can help reduce stress, promote relaxation, and relieve symptoms of digestive problems such as irritable bowel syndrome (IBS) and functional dyspepsia.

d. **Manual Therapies:** Chiropractic adjustments, osteopathic manipulation, and massage therapy can be used to treat musculoskeletal issues or promote relaxation, potentially benefiting people with functional dyspepsia or irritable bowel syndrome (IBS).

e. **Herbal Medicine:** Digestive issues can be treated with herbal medicines and botanical extracts in traditional medical systems such as Ayurveda or Western herbalism. Herbs such as chamomile, licorice root, slippery elm, and turmeric are thought to provide anti-inflammatory or digestive-supporting qualities.

Individuals with digestive issues must collaborate closely with healthcare practitioners to build a comprehensive treatment plan that addresses their unique requirements, preferences, and goals. Integrating conventional and alternative therapy options in a coordinated manner can result in a more comprehensive approach to controlling digestive issues and enhancing overall health. Individuals should also check with certified healthcare practitioners before beginning any new therapy or supplement regimen, particularly if they have pre-existing medical conditions or are on drugs.

Chapter 8: Dietary and Lifestyle Guidelines to Support Digestive Health

Dietary and lifestyle guidelines are essential for maintaining digestive health and controlling digestive problems. Here are some broad guidelines for improving digestive health:

Eat a balanced diet:

• Consume a range of nutrient-dense foods including fruits, vegetables, whole grains, lean meats, and healthy fats.

• Eat high-fiber foods like beans, lentils, nuts, seeds, whole grains, fruits, and vegetables to promote regular bowel movements and digestive health.

• Avoid processed foods, refined sugars, saturated fats, and high-fat foods, which can cause gastrointestinal discomfort and inflammation.

Stay hydrated:

• Drink lots of water all day to stay hydrated and promote healthy digestion.

• Limit your intake of caffeinated and alcoholic beverages, which can lead to dehydration and exacerbate stomach issues.

Eat mindfully:

• Practice mindful eating by observing hunger and fullness cues, chewing properly, and appreciating each bite.

• Avoid eating too quickly or when preoccupied, as this can result in overeating poor digestion, and gastrointestinal distress.

Manage portion sizes:

• Be cautious of portion amounts to avoid overeating and improve digestion.

• Aim for smaller, more frequent meals throughout the day to maintain energy and avoid intestinal pain.

Include probiotic foods:

• Include probiotic-rich foods in your diet, such as yogurt, kefir, sauerkraut, kimchi, miso, and kombucha, to promote a healthy gut microbiome and enhance digestion.

• Select fermented foods that contain living, active cultures of helpful bacteria.

Limit Trigger Foods:

• Identify and limit or avoid foods that cause digestive problems including acid reflux, bloating, gas, or diarrhea.

• Common trigger foods include spicy meals, fatty foods, coffee, alcohol, carbonated beverages, dairy products (for lactose intolerance), and certain high-fiber foods (for irritable bowel syndrome or other digestive disorders).

Manage stress:

• Use stress-reduction strategies such as deep breathing exercises, meditation, yoga, tai chi, or progressive muscle relaxation to induce relaxation and alleviate stress-related digestive issues.

• Set aside time for self-care, hobbies, and activities that promote relaxation and well-being.

Engage in regular physical activity:

• Include frequent physical activity to improve general health and bowel regularity.

• Try to get at least 30 minutes of moderate-intensity activity most days of the week, such as walking, swimming, cycling, or yoga.

Get Adequate Sleep:

• Make getting enough sleep a priority every night, since poor sleep quality and insufficient sleep can have a detrimental influence on digestion and overall health.

• Aim for 7-9 hours of sleep per night and follow a consistent sleep routine.

Seek professional guidance:

• Speak with a qualified dietitian or healthcare professional to receive specialized dietary and lifestyle recommendations based on your unique needs, preferences, and digestive health objectives.

• If you have a diagnosed digestive issue or are experiencing persistent or severe digestive symptoms, consult a gastroenterologist or other healthcare specialist.

Individuals who follow this dietary and lifestyle advice can enhance their digestive health, control digestive symptoms, and general well-being. Making modest modifications and determining what works best for your body can result in long-term digestive support and a healthier lifestyle.

Digestive-Friendly Recipes

Certainly! Here are a few simple and digestive-friendly dishes that use nutrient-dense ingredients and are soft on the stomach:

Quinoa and Vegetable Stir-Fry:

Ingredients:

1 cup quinoa, rinsed

2 cups water or vegetable broth

1 tablespoon olive oil

2 cloves garlic, minced

1 small onion, diced

2 cups of mixed veggies (bell peppers, broccoli, carrots, snap peas)

2 tablespoons low-sodium soy sauce or tamari

Salt and pepper to taste

Instructions:

• Heat water or vegetable broth in a medium pot until it boils. Add the quinoa, decrease the heat to low, cover, and simmer for 15-20 minutes, or until the quinoa is cooked and the water is absorbed.

• Prepare the olive oil in a large saucepan over medium heat. Sauté minced garlic and sliced onion until aromatic.

• Add the mixed vegetables to the skillet and stir-fry until soft and crisp.

• Add cooked quinoa and soy sauce, tossing until well blended. Add salt and pepper to taste.

• Serve hot, and enjoy!

Ginger-Turmeric Carrot Soup:

Ingredients:

1 tablespoon olive oil

1 small onion, diced

2 cloves garlic, minced

1 tablespoon fresh ginger, grated

1 tablespoon of freshly grated turmeric (or 1 teaspoon ground turmeric)

4 cups carrots, peeled and chopped

4 cups vegetable broth

Salt and pepper to taste

Fresh cilantro or parsley for garnish (optional)

Instructions:

• In a big pot, put the olive oil on a low heat. Combine the diced onion, minced garlic, grated ginger, and grated turmeric. Sauté till fragrant.

• Cook the chopped carrots for a few minutes.

• Bring the vegetable broth to a boil. Reduce the heat to low, cover, and cook for 20-25 minutes, until the carrots are soft.

• Using an immersion or countertop blender, puree the soup until smooth—season with salt and pepper to taste. Garnish with fresh cilantro or parsley as preferred. Serve hot, with a slice of whole-grain bread or crackers.

Baked Salmon with Lemon-Herb Quinoa:

Ingredients:

4 salmon fillets

2 tablespoons olive oil

1 tablespoon fresh lemon juice

1 teaspoon lemon zest

2 cloves garlic, minced

Salt and pepper to taste

1 cup quinoa, rinsed

2 cups water or vegetable broth

1 tablespoon fresh herbs (such as parsley, dill, or cilantro), chopped.

Instructions:

• Preheat the oven to 400°F (200°C). Arrange the salmon fillets on a baking pan lined with parchment paper.

• In a small bowl, combine the olive oil, lemon juice, lemon zest, minced garlic, salt, and pepper. Brush the mixture on the salmon fillets.

• Bake fish in a preheated oven for 12-15 minutes, or until thoroughly cooked and flaky.

• While the salmon bakes, make the quinoa. Heat water or vegetable broth in a medium pot until it boils. Add the quinoa, decrease the heat to low, cover, and simmer for 15-20 minutes, or until the quinoa is cooked and the water is absorbed.

• Fluff-cooked quinoa with a fork, then toss in fresh herbs.

• Serve baked fish with lemon-herb quinoa and steamed vegetables for a healthful and digestible supper.

These dishes are intended to be easy to digest while still providing important nutrients and flavors. Feel free to modify them according to your preferences and dietary requirements. Enjoy your meals!

Tips to Improve Digestive Health Naturally

Improving digestive health naturally entails adopting good lifestyle habits and eating foods that promote optimal digestion. Here are some strategies to improve digestive health naturally:

• **Maintain a Balanced Diet:** Eat a range of nutrient-dense foods, such as fruits, vegetables, whole grains, lean protein, and healthy fats. Consume fiber-rich meals including fruits, vegetables, legumes, and whole grains to promote bowel regularity and digestive health.

• **Stay Hydrated:** Drink plenty of water throughout the day to stay hydrated and encourage proper digestion. Limit your intake of caffeinated and alcoholic beverages, which can lead to dehydration and exacerbate stomach issues.

• **Include Probiotic Foods:** To maintain a healthy gut microbiome and enhance digestion, include probiotic-rich foods like yogurt, kefir, sauerkraut, kimchi, miso, and kombucha in your diet. These foods include helpful microorganisms that improve digestive health.

• **Manage Stress:** Deep breathing exercises, meditation, yoga, tai chi, or progressive muscle relaxation can all help you relax and lessen stress-related digestive issues. Chronic stress can impair digestive function, therefore managing stress is critical for overall digestive health.

• **Chew Your Food Thoroughly:** Take your time chewing and eating. Chewing food reduces it to smaller bits, making it easier to digest and absorb nutrients. Eating too fast or when distracted might result in overeating and poor digestion.

• **Limit Trigger Foods:** Identify and avoid foods that cause digestive problems including acid reflux, bloating, gas, or diarrhea. Spicy foods, fatty foods, caffeine, alcohol, carbonated beverages, dairy products (for those with lactose intolerance), and certain high-fiber foods (for those with irritable bowel syndrome or other digestive disorders) are all potential triggers.

• **Exercise Regularly:** Regular physical activity promotes general health and intestinal regularity. Aim for 30 minutes of moderate-intensity activity most days of the week, such as walking, swimming, cycling, or yoga. Exercise promotes digestion and relieves constipation.

• **Get Adequate Sleep:** Make getting enough sleep a priority every night, since poor sleep quality and insufficient sleep can have a detrimental influence on digestion and general well-being. Aim for 7-9 hours of sleep per night and follow a consistent sleep routine.

• **Limit Antibiotic Use:** Antibiotics should be used sparingly and only when required, as they can alter the balance of gut microbiota and cause gastrointestinal problems including diarrhea or dysbiosis. If you must take antibiotics, consider taking probiotic pills to help restore gut flora.

• **Seek Professional Help:** Speak with a registered dietitian or healthcare practitioner about specialized dietary and lifestyle suggestions based on your unique needs, preferences, and digestive health objectives. If you have been diagnosed with a digestive illness or are experiencing persistent or severe digestive symptoms, consult a gastroenterologist or healthcare professional.

By implementing these natural strategies into your daily routine, you can promote digestive health and general well-being. Making modest modifications and determining what works best for your body can result in long-term digestive support and a healthier lifestyle.

Conclusion

To summarize, empowering yourself for digestive wellness is adopting proactive measures to improve your digestive health through lifestyle changes, food choices, and self-care activities. Incorporate the following practices into your daily routine to optimize digestion, reduce symptoms, and promote overall well-being:

• **Healthy Eating Habits:** Follow a well-balanced diet rich in fruits, vegetables, whole grains, lean proteins, and healthy fats. Consume fiber-rich and probiotic-rich meals to maintain bowel regularity and a healthy gut microbiota.

• **Hydration:** stay hydrated by drinking plenty of water all day. Limit your intake of caffeinated and alcoholic beverages, which can lead to dehydration and exacerbate stomach issues.

• **Stress Management:** Use stress-reduction practices like deep breathing exercises, meditation, yoga, or mindfulness to improve relaxation and alleviate stress-related digestive issues.

• **Mindful Eating:** Eat slowly, chew carefully, and pay attention to hunger and fullness signals. Avoid eating fast or when preoccupied, as this might result in overeating and poor digestion.

• **Regular Exercise:** Exercise daily to help with digestion, enhance bowel regularity, and reduce stress. Aim for no less than 30 minutes of moderate-intensity exercise on most days of the week.

• **Sleep:** Prioritize getting enough sleep every night to improve overall health and digestion. Aim for 7-9 hours of sleep per night and follow a consistent sleep routine.

• **Limit Trigger Foods:** Identify and avoid foods that cause digestive problems including acid reflux, bloating, gas, or diarrhea. Spicy, greasy, caffeine, alcohol, and high-fiber diets are all potential triggers.

• **Seek Professional Help:** Speak with a qualified dietitian or healthcare practitioner about specialized dietary and lifestyle suggestions based on your specific needs and digestive health objectives. If you have been diagnosed with a digestive issue or are experiencing chronic or severe symptoms, consult a gastroenterologist or healthcare professional.

By taking control of your digestive health and applying these empowering tactics, you may improve digestive wellness, relieve discomfort, and improve your overall quality of life. Remember that even minor changes can have a major impact, and figuring out what works best for your body is essential for long-term digestive health.